MW01595977

CROHN'S
DISEASE

CROHN'S DISEASE

The Monster Uncovered

SHARON CATES

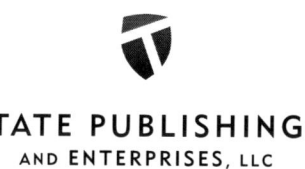

TATE PUBLISHING
AND ENTERPRISES, LLC

This book is designed to provide accurate and authoritative information with regard to the subject matter covered. This information is given with the understanding that neither the author nor Tate Publishing, LLC is engaged in rendering legal, professional advice. Since the details of your situation are fact dependent, you should additionally seek the services of a competent professional.

The opinions expressed by the author are not necessarily those of Tate Publishing, LLC.

Published by Tate Publishing & Enterprises, LLC
127 E. Trade Center Terrace | Mustang, Oklahoma 73064 USA
1.888.361.9473 | www.tatepublishing.com

Tate Publishing is committed to excellence in the publishing industry. The company reflects the philosophy established by the founders, based on Psalm 68:11,
"The Lord gave the word and great was the company of those who published it."

Published in the United States of America

ISBN: 978-1-61862-939-5
1. Self-Help / General
2. Health & Fitness / Diseases / Gastrointestinal
12.10.26

A MOTHER'S RESEARCH

HUNDREDS OF HOURS OF DOCUMENTED RESEARCH BY A MOTHER DESPERATELY SEARCHING TO CURE HER DAUGHTER OF CROHN'S DISEASE

Sharon M. Cates

ACKNOWLEDGMENTS

To my family, who inspire me to be a better daughter, sister, mother, grandmother, and friend, I love you all.

The author designed the information to represent her opinions about the subjects disclosed. The reader must weigh carefully all aspects of any medical decision before making any changes in his or her treatment. The author obtained the information contained through personal experience and research.

Disclaimer: the author disclaims any liability, loss, or risk incurred by individuals who act on the information contained herein. The author believes the advice presented here is sound, but readers cannot hold Sharon Cates responsible for either the actions they take or the results of those actions. The information provided throughout this book should not be used for diagnosing or treating Crohn's disease without consulting your health care provider. This information is not a substitute for professional care.

TABLE OF CONTENTS

FIRST DIAGNOSED

To all those diagnosed with any stage of Crohn's disease, I know you most likely feel overwhelmed just as I felt after hearing my daughter's heartrending diagnosis.

MY STORY

Test results confirmed what we feared: Crohn's disease.

My daughter, Kelly, was only nineteen years old when she was diagnosed with Crohn's disease. Prior to her diagnosis, she was a young woman attending the University of Kentucky working towards her dreams of becoming an attorney. During Kelly's second year of studies, she became ill with recurring stomach aches, diarrhea, and high fevers. The campus doctor's conclusion was that stress was causing Kelly to be sick. Unable to cope any longer, Kelly finished her second year, then dropped out of school and came home to de-stress and get healthy. Regardless of Kelly's strong will, her health became progressively worse, and it was only one month after Kelly came home that she was diagnosed with having ulcerative colitis. Her doctor prescribed corticosteroids for the inflammation and Lortab for the pain.

Eight weeks and three emergency room trips later, another colonoscopy confirmed full-blown Crohn's disease. At that time, we knew very little about this horrible disease. We discussed aggressive treatments and a cure with Kelly's gastroenterologist. Imagine my shock to hear there was no cure and that my sweet Kelly had been sentenced to a lifelong battle with a monster named Crohn's. The doctor started Kelly on a regimen of steroids, antibiotics, and stronger pain medication, with a scheduled colonoscopy to follow-up in six months.

That day seemed like a nightmare to me. I felt as if a ton of bricks had dropped onto me as I listened to the doctor telling us to prepare ourselves for a long battle and possibly surgery. He went so far as to strongly recommend that Kelly sign up for disability as her ability to hold a job with this diagnosis would be nearly impossible. We were devastated to say the very least and left the doctor's office crying for what seemed to be a long, dismal future for Kelly fighting a hopeless battle.

Like any parent, I listened and heard what the doctors had to say, and perhaps I was in denial, but I would not accept such a hopeless diagnosis. I started researching this monster disease, looking for the causes, the treatments, alternative treatments, and mostly, a cure.

Did I find that cure? *Yes.* I not only found the product that cured my daughter, she has been symptom free, and more importantly drug free, for over ten years now. As a matter of fact, Kelly's gastroenterologist was amazed at the results of that scheduled six-month follow-up colonoscopy. In his own words, "It's a miracle, no signs of Crohn's, only a pink, perfectly healthy colon. There is no way to explain this other than a miracle."

Kelly did at that time confess that she had turned to an alternative treatment and had stopped taking his prescribed meds two months earlier. She handed him a pamphlet that she had brought along describing the alternative treatment she had been using. Her hope was that he would pass the word and this alternative treatment would help other Crohn's patients as it had for her. There was no doubt that he was astonished at the test results: "A miracle, just a miracle," he kept repeating. He admitted that he had never seen anyone turn severe Crohn's Disease around like she had; however, he could not suggest to other Crohn's sufferers this alternative treatment. He claimed that this product had not been approved by the Food and Drug Administration; therefore, as a physician, he could not recommend the use of this alternative treatment to other Crohn's patients. He handed Kelly back the pamphlet with little more to say on the subject.

Kelly was disappointed with what seemed to be her doctor's uncaring position for others suffering this same horrible disease. As for me, I was just happy that Kelly had reclaimed her life from the horrible beast, Crohn's.

Recently, while watching a local news broadcast on the topic "Weight Gain and The Effects of Medications," I realized the lack of movement in treating Crohn's disease. Interviewed on that broadcast was a young woman who had gained over fifteen pounds since being diagnosed with Crohn's disease and prescribed a regimen of strong steroids. I could see the anxiety in her eyes and knew in that moment that I had to share my research with others suffering with this horrible disease. I felt compelled to make my research available to others who might be looking for information and alternative treatment options like the one that vanquished this monster disease from my daughter, saving her from a lifetime of pain and suffering.

Keep in mind that I am not a doctor, but rather I am a caring mother who spent countless hours researching Crohn's disease. That research is what I am sharing with you—the causes, statistics, medical treatments, alternative treatments, and how to survive with Crohn's. I hope you find this research to be helpful in educating yourself about the disease and available treatment options.

A MOTHERS RESEARCH

THE MONSTER UNCOVERED

CROHN'S DISEASE

Crohn's Disease is a chronic inflammatory bowel disease that causes an inflammation of the digestive tract. While Crohn's disease primarily involves the small and large intestines, it can affect other parts of the digestive system. There are five different types of Crohn's disease.

Types of Crohn's Disease

- Ileitis affects only the small intestines (ileum).
- Jejunoileitis Crohn's causes spotty patches of inflammation in the top half of the small intestine (jejunum).
- Ileocolitis is the most common form of Crohn's and affects the lowest part of the small intestine (ileum) and the large intestine (colon).
- Crohn's Colitis (granulomatous) affects only the large intestine.

- Gastroduodenal, the least common of Crohn's diseases, causes inflammation in the stomach and first part of the small intestine called the duodenum.

Crohn's disease was first described by doctors as a bowel disease in 1932.

STATISTICS

Though Crohn's disease can occur at any point in life, the disease is usually diagnosed in persons between the ages of fifteen and thirty-five. Men and women are at equal risk. To my surprise, roughly 20 percent of people with Crohn's disease have a sibling, parent, or child with some form of bowel disease. According to the National Institute of Allergy and Infectious Diseases (NIAID), a division of the US Department of Health and Human Services, approximately one in five hundred people suffer from inflammatory bowel disease. The National Institute of Diabetes & Digestive & Kidney Diseases (NIDDK) reports similar numbers with approximately 544,000 people suffering with bowel diseases in the United States. Approximately fifty-four thousand of those are under the age of eighteen. Approximately 700,000 doctor's office visits are attributed to inflammatory bowel disease annually. Doctor's visits and hospital stays cost Americans who suffer from these digestive diseases an estimated $87 billion annually. Another $20 billion is spent on indirect medical costs, which include disability and mortality.

The statistics for persons with Crohn's disease receiving Social Security Disability Insurance is estimated at 119,000 Americans. In Europe, concerns about appropriate treatment for Crohn's disease led to a study in which ten gastroenterologists, three surgeons, and two general practitioners from twelve different countries evaluated their colleagues' treatment of Crohn's disease patients. The results were not good. The panel found that treatment was inappropriate an alarming 52 percent of the time. After evaluating the statistics for Crohn's disease treatment, this expert panel came up with a set of guidelines that is used today to help practitioners treat patents in what was deemed an appropriate manner.

These treatments include medications that are anti-inflammatory, immune suppressors, antibiotics, and surgery in severe cases. The Department of Gastroenterology in London reported that the use of complementary and alternative medicine for the treatment of Crohn's syndrome and ulcerative colitis, particularly herbal therapies, was widespread and on the increase. According to this study, there was evidence that aloe and acupuncture were promising and might be effective in reducing inflammation and pain associated with inflammatory bowel disease.

So what happened to further studies on herbal therapies? Well, the panel was concerned that certain herbal preparations may interact with prescription medications and, if not used under doctor's supervision, would not be safe. They were also concerned with the quality of products that patients might receive.

It is due to these concerns the statistics for Crohn's disease treatment with herbal and alternative therapies relating to effectiveness, side effects, cures, and safety are unavailable as no further surveys or studies were done at that time.

I found this reasoning to be very disturbing. Are natural remedies and cures being censored and hidden from us just because greedy health-care professionals, pharmaceutical companies, and hospitals want to make more money? It is my personal opinion that because Crohn's disease is not considered a life threatening disease and only affects one's quality of life, we are led to believe there is no cure and that the real reason there are no studies on herbal alternatives is solely the financial hit that doctors, hospitals, and pharmaceutical companies would suffer if Crohn's patients could be cured with low cost herbal remedies. Any herbal alternative study with a positive outcome would most definitely interfere with this multi-billion dollar disease.

Well, I say that if there is an herbal alternative that cures or even lessens the horrible side effects of Crohn's disease, we, the people, deserve to know.

A CROHN'S QUIZ TO TEST YOUR KNOWLEDGE

When it comes to Crohn's disease information, can you separate fact from fiction? With all the Crohn's information available on the internet, it's hard to know what to believe sometimes. Take the quiz below and get the truth to some of the most frequently asked questions.

> **Q.** Eating certain foods can cause Crohn's disease. True or False?
>
> **A.** False—There is no evidence that eating certain foods causes Crohn's disease. However, once you have Crohn's, eating certain foods can worsen your symptoms, so it is important to make the right food choices. Consider talking with a dietitian.

> **Q.** Stress causes Crohn's disease. True or False?
>
> **A.** False—even though emotional stress may aggravate Crohn's disease, there is no evidence that stress causes Crohn's disease. In fact, it's more likely that it's the other way around. Living with a long-term condition like Crohn's can cause a range of emotions including stress.

Q. There is no cure for Crohn's disease. True or False?

A. True—there is no Food & Drug Administration-approved medication known to cure Crohn's Disease.

Q. Crohn's disease is contagious. True or False?

A. False—Crohn's disease is not contagious. A person with Crohn's cannot give the condition to someone else, no matter how much contact people have with others.

Q. Crohn's disease can cause minimal symptoms with or even without medical treatment? True or False?

A. True—Crohn's disease symptoms may range from a chronic, recurrent condition to very mild with minimal symptoms.

Q. Crohn's disease symptoms are solely associated with the digestive tract? True or False?

A. False—Crohn's disease can also be associated with reddish skin nodules and inflammation of the joints, spine, eyes, and liver.

Q. Doctors use inflammatory drugs to cure Crohn's disease? True or False

A. False—inflammatory drug treatment for Crohn's disease is aimed at controlling Crohn's symptoms.

Q. If you are having bouts with diarrhea, vomiting, and fever. it is a good idea to wait a few weeks before contacting a doctor. True or False?

A. False—early diagnosis and early treatment is your best defense in preventing Crohn's complications.

SYMPTOMS

Symptoms depend on what part of the gastrointestinal tract is affected. Symptoms range from mild to severe with periods of flare-ups that come and go.

The more common symptoms of Crohn's disease are:

- Abdominal cramping in the belly area
- Fever
- Fatigue
- Loss of appetite
- Pain with passing stool
- Persistent, watery diarrhea
- Unintentional weight loss

More severe symptoms from ongoing flare-ups include:

- Severe Constipation
- Frequent hospitalization
- Stunted growth in adolescents
- Eye inflammation
- Fistulas or small tears usually around the rectal area
- Joint pain
- Excessive weight loss
- Liver inflammation
- Mouth ulcers
- Rectal bleeding and bloody stools
- Skin rash
- Swollen gums

CAUSE AND EFFECT

While the exact cause of Crohn's disease is unknown, the condition is linked to a problem with the body's immune system response. Normally, the immune system helps protect the body, but with Crohn's disease, the immune system cannot tell the difference between normal body tissue and foreign substances. The result is an overactive immune response that leads to chronic inflammation. The medical term for this overactive immune system is autoimmune disorder. Your immune system is unable to recognize normal, good proteins brought into the body through blood, bacteria, and food. The result is your own immune system declares war on your body.

In an effort to combat what usually are normal proteins, the turned-on immune system is altered, treating normal proteins and nutrients in the digestive tract as dangerous. The immune system then sends excessive white blood cells to the inner walls of the colon, leading to the formation of ulcers.

In serious cases, deeper and larger ulcers can develop, causing scarring and possibly narrowing of the bowel, which sometimes leads to an obstruction in the bowel. These large ulcers can progress deep into the wall of the bowel, causing puncture holes and resulting in infection of the abdominal cavity and in adjacent organs. In acute cases, surgery might be needed if the inflammation has caused permanent intestinal damage that cannot be repaired.

It is the abnormality in the immune system that researchers feel is the foremost cause of Crohn's disease, rather than any external cause. However, other researched causes appear to be a result of a complex interaction of factors including:

- Inherited genes
- A weak immune system
- Environmental factors
- A family history of Crohn's disease

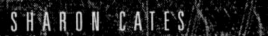
- Jewish ancestry
- Smoking

WHEN SHOULD YOU CONTACT YOUR DOCTOR

It is strongly suggested that you call for an appointment with your trained health care provider if:

- You have symptoms of Crohn's disease.
- You are already diagnosed with Crohn's disease and your symptoms get worse or do not improve with treatment.
- You are already diagnosed with Crohn's disease and you develop new symptoms.

Your best defense is to be diagnosed early and start treatment early to prevent complications. Inflammation that goes on for long periods of time without being diagnosed can be dangerous.

DIAGNOSING CROHN'S DISEASE

The diagnosis of any form of inflammatory colon disorder is directed by the symptoms of abdominal pain, rectal bleeding, and diarrhea. Diagnosing involves taking blood and stool samples, followed by imaging and internal inspection.

Most often, a blood report is first used to rule out the infectious and parasitic causes of diarrhea such as those caused by food poisoning. This blood report is also used to detect whether or not you have developed anemia due to the passing of blood through the stool. Stool samples are obtained and examined for presence of blood cells. If these initial tests indicate a form of inflammatory bowel disease, most doctors will order an X-ray or an ultrasound scan of the lower abdomen before ordering an internal inspection. Images will show the inflamed area quite well and can partially confirm the presence and stage of inflammatory bowel disease. Once it is confirmed that inflammatory bowel disease is present, your doctor will usually then refer you to a gastroenterologist experienced in bowel disease treatment.

Tests can be scary, so the more you know about the tests before hand, the less stressful it will be. Below are a list of tests and procedures that your doctors may order to help in diagnosing Crohn's disease and its severity:

- Blood Test—a laboratory analysis performed on a blood sample that is usually extracted from a vein in the arm using a needle. The blood will be analyzed for anemia, a condition that may point to bleeding in the intestines, and to elevated white blood cell count, which is a sign of inflammation in the colon.
- Stool specimens are collected for analysis to test for blood in your stool. Stool analysis will also exclude

infection and parasites, since these conditions can cause symptoms that mimic Crohn's disease.

- An ultrasound scan is a painless test that uses sound waves to create images of the abdomen. Ultrasound scanning may help rule in or rule out Crohn's disease, but further X-ray validation will required if the ultrasound scan suggests Crohn's.

- Computed Tomography (CT) Scan uses X-rays to make detailed images inside the abdomen. During the test you will lie on a table that is attached to a large doughnut shaped machine. An iodine dye is often used to make structures and organs easier to see on the CT image. The dye may be administered through a vein in your arm or directly into the rectum.

- An endoscope is an instrument with a light attached used to examine the interior of hollow organs or cavities of the body. The most common endoscopy used to diagnose Crohn's disease is the colonoscopy. The colonoscopy allows direct visualization of the interior lining of the colon and rectum using a thin flexible tube with an attached camera. This visualization will establish the diagnosis and help in determining the severity of your colitis. During the procedure your gastroenterologist might also perform a biopsy, taking small samples of the diseased tissue for laboratory analysis, which will be helpful in confirmation and treatment options. If you have signs and symptoms that suggest Crohn's disease but other diagnostic tests are negative, your doctor may perform a capsule endoscopy. For this test you will swallow a capsule that has a tiny camera in it. The camera takes pictures, which are transmitted to a computer that you will wear on your belt. The images are then downloaded and displayed on a monitor, checking for Crohn's disease. Once the capsule has made the trip through your digestive system, the camera exits your body painlessly in your stool. While the capsule endoscopy offers a very high accuracy, it is limited by the inability to obtain biopsies. Discuss with your gastroenterologist which endoscopy procedure is best for you. Keep in mind that knowledge of the extent and severity of Crohn's disease is essential in choosing your treatment options.

- Magnetic Resonance Imaging (MRI) of the abdomen is useful in evaluating Crohn's disease of the small intestine, because a colonoscopy cannot not be used to evaluate the entire small intestine. MRI scans are also useful in detecting abnormal complications of Crohn's disease, such as abscesses, small bowel obstructions, or small tears in the intestines.

- A barium enema X-ray may also indicate a diagnosis of Crohn's. During a barium enema, a chalky dye substance containing barium is administered into the rectum and into the colon. Barium is radiopaque and can outline the colon on x-ray pictures. A barium enema is less accurate and useful than direct visualization techniques in the diagnosis of Crohn's disease.

- Upper GI series consist of a series of X-ray images of the esophagus, stomach, and small intestines. Because Crohn's disease can be found throughout the digestive tract from the mouth to the rectum, an upper GI series of X-rays will determine if Crohn's disease is present in the esophagus, stomach, or small intestines. In this procedure, a chalky radiopaque contrast is drunk, allowing X-ray images of these areas to be made.

LIVING WITH CROHN'S DISEASE: PRACTICAL STRATEGIES

Now that you have been diagnosed with Crohn's Disease, what is the next step? By now you are most likely feeling overwhelmed and not sure what to do. You might be thinking, *Should I get another medical opinion? What is my life going to be like? What about all the medicines the doctor wants me to take, are they safe? Are there other treatments available, that he has not mentioned?*

Let's start with what your life is going to be like with Crohn's Disease and continue from there.

LIFE

Not knowing whether your life expectancy is going to be shorter when you have Crohn's disease is a very real concern until you find the answers. The good news is that people with Crohn's disease have a relatively normal life span, and while Crohn's disease can be very scary, you don't need to be worried about your life expectancy. There is no reason why you won't live to a ripe old age and enjoy all the great things that life has to offer the same as everyone else.

Most Crohn's patients experience flare ups followed by episodes of remission when the symptoms decrease or even disappear. Since there have been major improvements in the recognition and management of Crohn's in the last fifty years, the risk of major complications or death during the severest attacks of Crohn's Disease have fallen below 3 percent.

Natural treatments also have come a long way; it is now possible to easily control your Crohn's Disease naturally. Using such things as diet, exercise, herbal therapy, and stress-controlling techniques can give you some control over your flare-ups.

EDUCATE YOURSELF

Before your next doctor's visit, write down your questions to make sure you don't leave any concerns unanswered. You can also ask a relative or friend to come with you to your appointments to make sure you remember everything your doctor has said.

As you learn more about your condition, you may hear about men and women who have had a hard time coping with their illness. Reading about these stories may make you feel hopeless. It's very important to realize that no two people experience Crohn's disease in the same way. Just because some people have a severe form of the disease doesn't mean that you will. Instead, try to focus on learning all that you can to manage your condition.

TALK WITH FAMILY AND FRIENDS

Not everyone is comfortable sharing the fact that they have a serious health condition. But doing so can ease the extra stress of trying to hide it. Explain Crohn's disease in a matter-of-fact way—that it can cause attacks of pain and diarrhea. This will help those close to you understand why you often need to use the bathroom or don't feel up to socializing. Letting family and friends know what you are going through also means that you can turn to them for support and reassurance. They can be there for you during disease flares when you need extra help with grocery shopping or child care or need a ride to doctor's appointments.

You may also want to consider talking with your supervisor at work and trusted co-workers about your condition. This will go a long way toward explaining extended absences at work and frequent bathroom breaks. Read up on the Family and Medical Leave Act (FMLA) so that you know your rights in the event that you need to take off work for an extended period of time.

PLAN YOUR EVERY DAY

The unpredictable nature of some symptoms, such as diarrhea, gas, and abdominal pain may discourage you from leading an active life. However, it's important to make efforts to participate in the activities you enjoyed before your diagnosis and to maintain your daily life as normally as possible.

Here are some planning tips that may help you:

- Choosing familiar destinations may be a good starting point. Once you feel more comfortable, you might try less familiar places.
- Discreetly noting the location of bathrooms on or before arrival is not only practical, but it also may help minimize your stress.
- You also may find it helpful to travel with extra toilet tissue and undergarments.

REDUCE STRESS IN YOUR LIFE

As with diet, stress does not cause the onset of Crohn's disease, but stress still plays an important role for many Crohn's patients, often prompting flare-ups and aggravating symptoms. Pay attention to your body. If stress causes added problems for you, try some of the following techniques to help you manage your stress levels:

- Try progressive relaxation exercises like yoga, meditation, or deep breathing.
- Exercise regularly to reduce stress levels and aid in normal bowel function. Consult your doctor before beginning any exercise regimen.
- In some instances, people with Crohn's disease may benefit from some form of counseling. Your healthcare provider may refer you to a suitable therapist.

CREATE YOUR SUPPORT SYSTEM

Joining a support group can provide you with the kind of help you can only get from people who know what you are going through.

Communicating positively with others may reduce the emotional impact of Crohn's disease and make the adjustment easier for you. In addition, an honest and open relationship with your healthcare provider may help ensure you receive the best possible care.

Persons with Crohn's disease often find it comforting to connect with others undergoing similar experiences. Support groups may provide you with a safe and constructive emotional outlet and practical strategies to cope with the broad impact of your disease. To find a support group in your area visit the Crohn's & Colitis Foundation of America (CCFA) website, www.ccfa.org

Another way to gain the support you need in managing your condition is to join the Crohn's & Colitis Community, www.ccfacommunity.org. As a member of this free, online community, you'll be able to talk to others suffering with Crohn's disease through online discussion boards and forums. You can share your personal story and read other members' stories. Remember, one in five people have some form of inflammatory bowel syndrome; there is no reason to suffer alone. A positive support system can go a long way in helping you to manage your flare-ups.

CHOOSE YOUR DIET CAREFULLY

Although there is no evidence that diet is a direct cause of Crohn's disease, the foods you eat might make a difference in the severity of your symptoms. For instance, you may find that certain foods and beverages are less tolerable during flare-ups. While everyone is different, some of the foods that are commonly less tolerable include:

- Dairy products
- Spicy foods

- Some foods high in fiber
- Some foods high in fat

Keep a personal food journal to help manage your symptoms. As you begin your Crohn's treatment, take note of the symptoms you have and when. Do you always have diarrhea after eating? Are symptoms usually more active at a specific time of day? By recognizing when you are more likely to have symptoms, you can plan your day around them. Also note which, if any, foods affect your bowel problems. Many people with Crohn's disease find they need to avoid high-fiber foods such as seeds, nuts, popcorn, and corn, as well as spicy, fried, and greasy foods.

You may want to talk with your doctor about working with a registered dietitian (RD). He or she can review your food diary to determine whether you are eating a balanced diet. An RD can help you plan meals so that you get a wide range of nutritious foods. Eliminating and reintroducing certain components of your diet may be a useful technique in learning about your food sensitivities. Another dietary concern for you will be poor nutrition because of the poor absorption and loss of appetite often associated with the disease.

PLAN YOUR TRIPS

The classic symptoms of Crohn's disease—persistent diarrhea, pain, and cramping—can make you feel hesitant to stray very far from home. That's understandable early on when you are learning how your condition affects you. But don't get into the habit of cutting yourself off from the rest of the world. Planning ahead can help give you a sense of security so that you can go about your daily routine as much as possible.

Locate restrooms in public areas such as restaurants, shopping malls, highway rest areas, and anywhere you tend to go in your local area. This can help you keep a mental map of bathroom stops in mind when you are out and about. There is even an application for some handheld devices that can help you locate restrooms in your area.

Pack a travel kit that includes a spare set of underwear, toilet tissue, wipes, a couple of zip-top bags, and deodorizer. You may never need it, but just knowing it's there if you do have an accident can help give you peace of mind. Ask a trusted friend to be on-call to come get you should you find yourself in a difficult situation.

FOCUS ON YOUR FUTURE

The fact that you have been diagnosed with Crohn's disease may be all you can think about now. But it won't always be that way. Keep your focus on your future and remember: having Crohn's disease does not have to control your life.

YOUR TREATMENT

FINDING THE RIGHT TREATMENT FOR YOU

Because the type, symptoms, and severity of Crohn's disease can differ from person to person, treatment will also differ, as well. What's right for one person might not be right for you. Work with your doctor to learn as much as you can about Crohn's disease treatment options, and find the treatment that meets your individual needs. And don't wait—the sooner you and your doctor identify a treatment plan, the sooner you will be able to start controlling your symptoms.

DIET AND NUTRITION

I want to touch once again on the importance of diet and nutrition in relation to your treatment. A nutritious diet is very helpful during treatment, and eating a healthy amount of calories, vitamins, and protein is important to avoid malnutrition, weight loss, and severe complications. Certain types of foods may worsen diarrhea and gas symptoms, especially during times of active disease. Know how the foods you are eating are affecting your treatment.

Suggestions for diet during periods when symptoms are present include:

- Eat small amounts of food throughout the day.
- Drink lots of water—frequent consumption of small amounts throughout the day.
- Avoid high-fiber foods—bran, beans, nuts, seeds, and popcorn.
- Avoid fatty, greasy, or fried foods and sauces like butter, margarine, and heavy cream.
- Avoid milk and dairy products.
- Avoid or limit alcohol and caffeine consumption.
- Avoid or limit spicy foods.
- Avoid raw fruits and vegetables if you have a blockage of the intestines.
- Stop smoking. Smoking may amplify Crohn's disease.

Discuss with your doctor extra vitamins and minerals you may need to help you fight Crohn's disease such as:

- Iron supplements (if you are anemic)
- Calcium and vitamin D supplements to help keep your bones strong
- Vitamin B-12 to prevent anemia

MEDICATIONS

According to medical journals, Crohn's is a lifelong condition, but there are prescription medications available. Even though there is no proven cure for Crohn's disease, there are medicines available to help control your symptoms. Crohn's treatment plans should be based on a person's individual needs. Keep in mind that your doctor's main goal in treating Crohn's disease is controlling inflammation, achieving remission, and maintaining remission. Work together with your doctor to find a treatment plan that helps you reach your treatment goals. Make sure you share how medications are affecting you and ask about any new treatment options.

There are 5 basic categories of prescription medications available to treat Crohn's disease:

- Mesalazine, also known as 5-aminosalicylic (5-ASAs), help control mild to moderate inflammation. Some forms of the drug are taken by mouth; others must be given rectally.
- Corticosteroids (prednisone and methylprednisolone) are used to treat moderate to severe Crohn's symptoms. They may be taken by mouth or by rectal steroids.

- Immune system suppressors reduce inflammation by targeting the immune system's reaction. They help reduce the need for corticosteroids.
- Antibiotics may be prescribed for abscesses or fistulas.
- Biologic therapy is used to treat patients with severe Crohn's disease that do not respond to any other types of medication. Medicines in this group include infliximab (Remicade) and adalimumab (Humira), certolizumab (Cimzia), and natalizumab (Tysabri). They belong to a class of drugs called monoclonal antibodies, which help block an immune system chemical that promotes inflammation.

PRESCRIPTION MEDICATIONS— PURPOSE & SIDE EFFECTS

Mesalazine

Mesalazine in an anti-inflammatory drug used to treat mild to moderate inflammation of the digestive tract caused by Crohn's disease. Mesalazine is bowel specific and acts locally in the gut. It is formulated for oral ingestion as tablets and for rectal administration as a suppository. One of the newest Mesalazine drugs to be approved by the US Food and Drug

Administration is Apriso. Other Mesalazine drugs are Asacol, Ipocal, Pentasa, Salofalk, Mezavant XL, Canasa, Rowasa, Pentasa, Lidalda, and Mesacol. The primary difference between these drug names is the mesalazine dose per tablet. Lialda contains the highest dose per tablet and Aprisco and Asacol contain some of the lowest dosage of mesalamine. It is believed that the Mesalazine drug in lower doses helps with maintenance of remission in Crohn's disease. As a result of the rare side effects and risk to the kidneys and liver, blood tests should be taken before and after starting treatment.

Common side effects include:

- Diarrhea
- Nausea
- Cramping

Some uncommon side effects include:

- Headache
- Hair Loss
- Rash or hives
- Sore throat
- Fever
- Bruising

Rare side effects include:

- Hepatitis
- Accute Pancreatitis
- Blood disorders

It is not uncommon for doctors to prescribe Mesalazine drugs along with corticosteroids.

Corticosteroids

Corticosteroids have been used for many years in the treatment of patients with moderate to severe Crohn's disease. Unlike the mesalazine compounds, corticosteroids do not require direct contact with the inflamed intestinal tissues to be effective. Oral corticosteroids are potent anti-inflammatory agents. After absorption, corticosteroids exert prompt anti-inflammatory action throughout the body. In critically ill patients, intravenous corticosteroids can be given in the hospital.

Corticosteroids are fast acting and patients frequently experience improvement in their symptoms within days of starting corticosteroids. Corticosteroids, however, do not work for everyone with Crohn's disease and are not for long term use due to the numerous potentially serious side effects. Short term use of Corticosteroids (three to four months) can improve symptoms and induce remission. Side effects of corticosteroids depend on the dose and duration of use. Short courses of prednisone, for example, usually are well tolerated with few and mild side effects. Long term, high doses of corticosteroids usually produce predictable and potentially serious side effects.

Common side effects include:

- Puffy face
- Excessive facial hair
- Night sweats
- Insomnia
- Weight gain
- High blood pressure
- Acne
- Depression

Serious side effects may occur and can include:

- Bone fractures
- Cataracts
- Susceptibility to infections
- Osteoporosis
- Muscle weakness
- Diabetes
- Stunted growth in children

Long term use may cause other serious side effects such as:

- Death of bone tissue of the hip joints
- Depressed adrenal glands
- Shock
- Withdrawal symptoms if corticosteroids are stopped too quickly. Corticosteroids need to be gradually reduced rather than abruptly stopped.

Because corticosteroids are not useful in maintaining remission in Crohn's disease and because they have predictable and potentially serious side effects, these drugs should be used for the shortest possible length of time. Once the symptoms are under control, the reduction of corticosteroids should occur at a slow pace. Some patients become corticosteroid dependent. In patients who are corticosteroid dependent or who are unresponsive to corticosteroids, other anti-inflammatory medications, immune system suppressors, should be considered.

Immune System Suppressors

Immune system suppressors are drugs that also reduce inflammation by targeting the immune system rather than directly treating inflammation as with corticosteroids. Immune system suppressors can also help maintain remission. The US Food and Drug Administration has approved the use of immunosuppressant drugs including: Azathioprine, mercaptopurine, methotrexate, imfliximab, adalimumab, certoilizumanb, cyclosporine, and natalizumab. Each of these drugs target the immune system to reduce inflammation; however, each has their own potency and specific immune system target. Each also has their own potential for serious side effects.

Potential common side effects include:

- Headache
- Upper respiratory infections
- Abdominal pain
- Nausea
- Diarrhea
- Fatigue

Potential serious side effects include:

- Fatal infections
- Kidney damage
- Liver damage
- Increased risk of cancer
- High blood pressure
- Seizures
- Brain infection

Antibiotics

Antibiotics may be used to control the infections caused by abscesses in the colon walls or fistulas. Researchers also believe antibiotics help reduce harmful intestinal bacteria and suppress the intestine's immune system. Antibiotics frequently prescribed for Crohn's patients are Metronidazole and Ciprofloxacin. Like other pharmaceutical medicines, antibiotics can have potentially serious side effects after periods of prolonged use.

Common side effects may include:

- Nausea
- Vomiting
- Headache

Potentially serious side effects can include:

- Tendon problems
- Muscle pain
- Muscle weakness
- Numbness in hands or feet

Biologic Therapy

Biologic therapy is used to treat patients with severe Crohn's disease that do not respond to any other Crohn's medications and treatments. A variety of biological therapies have been developed to treat Crohn's disease. Medicines in this group include Infliximab, Adalimumab, Certolizumab, and Natalizumab. They belong to a class of drugs called monoclonal antibodies, which help block an immune system chemical that promotes inflammation. This aggressive therapy should be closely monitored by medical professionals as the side effects associated with biologic therapy may be life-threatening.

Serious side effects may occur and can include:

- Risk of allergic reactions
- Reactivation of old infections like tuberculosis
- Later complications with onset of multiple sclerosis and lymphoma

OTHER MEDICATIONS

Some other medications that may help to relieve the symptoms of Crohn's disease include anti-diarrheals, laxatives, pain relievers, iron supplements, vitamin B-12 shots, calcium and vitamin D supplements.

CROHN'S COMPLICATIONS

In addition to the effects on the gastrointestinal tract, Crohn's disease can lead to many complications, including an obstruction of the intestine due to swelling and the formation of scar tissue. Other potential severe complications of Crohn's disease include malnutrition, the development of fissures (small cuts or tears in the anal canal), abscesses (localized infections or collections of pus), and fistulas (an abnormal tunnel that forms between two structures of the body). Patients suffering with blood loss from the inflamed intestines can lead to anemia and may require treatment with iron supplements or even blood transfusions. Rarely, the colon can acutely dilate to a large size when the inflammation becomes very severe. This condition is called toxic megacolon. Patients with toxic megacolon become extremely ill with fever, abdominal pain and distention, dehydration, and malnutrition. Unless the patient improves rapidly with medication, surgery usually is necessary to prevent colon rupture.

Complications of Crohn's disease can involve other parts of the body. Ten percent of patients can develop arthritis or mild inflammation of the joints. Rarely, patients may develop painful red skin nodules. Yet others can have painful red eyes. Diseases of the liver and bile ducts may also be associated with Crohn's disease.

Colon cancer is a recognized complication of chronic Crohn's disease and the risk for cancer begins to rise after eight to ten years of the onset of Crohn's disease. Patients at higher risk of cancer are patients with positive family histories of colon cancer, long durations of Crohn's disease, and extensive colon involvement. Since colon cancers have a more favorable outcome when diagnosed and treated at an earlier stage, yearly colon examinations may be recommended. During these examinations, samples of tissue (biopsies) can be taken to search for precancerous changes in the lining cells of the colon. When precancerous changes are found, removal of the colon may be necessary to prevent colon cancer.

SURGERY

For a few patients, surgery may be recommended at some point as a part of the therapeutic management. Surgery may be needed to clear an intestinal blockage, repair damage to the intestines, or treat symptoms that medication alone could not control. In severe cases, surgery may be needed to remove part of the colon. An external pouch then needs to be attached to collect and remove waste by a small opening surgically crafted in the lower abdomen. Another approach has the colon removed and a pouch created internally that connects the small intestine with the muscles in the anus. This way, patients can pass stool normally and bowel integrity is preserved as well.

For Crohn's patients, the benefits of surgery are only temporary as the disease most often recurs with more severe complications. Surgery may be considered when there are complications such as:

- Excessive bleeding (hemorrhage).
- Fistulas, the abnormal connections between the intestines and another area of the body.
- Sever life-threatening infections.
- Full or partial intestinal blockage.

ALTERNATIVE TREATMENTS

With the serious side effects of pharmaceutical treatments, it is no surprise that more than half of Crohn's disease sufferers have tried complementary or alternative therapy. Understand that when you have serious health conditions like Crohn's disease, it's important to seek medical attention, and your doctor should be your first resource to all current treatment options available.

ALTERNATIVE TREATMENTS RESEARCHED

Because of what seemed to be a hopeless diagnosis and the side effects that the medicines were having on my daughter, I started searching for alternative medicine to help her. One of the main characteristics we were looking for was that any alternative treatment could not interfere with the prescription medicines that her doctors had prescribed. As bad as the sided effects were, prescription medicines were the only hope provided by her gastroenterologist.

After many, many hours of researching alternative treatments for Crohn's disease, we selected one that both Kelly and I felt would be the best solution for her.

During my research, the one alternative treatment that repeatedly came up was the use of aloe in treating irritable bowel symptoms. While aloe in its pure form was not recommended for Crohn's suffers due to the fact that it has been found to amplify some of the common symptoms of Crohn's disease—diarrhea and stomach pain—other forms of aloe might be the answer.

A leading agronomist mastered a technique of processing the aloe plant from its purest form into a highly concentrated form of AMP or Aloe Mucilaginous Polysaccharide molecules, retaining the natural molecular structure of the long chain of polysaccharides found in the fresh, unprocessed aloe leaves. Simply clarified, you most likely have heard about the healing properties of aloe or the aloe vera plant, so that covers the *Aloe* part. The clear goo substance found inside the aloe leaf is *Mucilaginous*, simply meaning *sticky* and the word *Polysaccharide* is a combination of *poly* meaning many and sugars. So by definition, AMPs are long chains of sugar molecules, made up of individual sugar molecules connected together in a sticky substance, with the ability to regulate the body's immune system to a natural healthy level. This is a major breakthrough for uses of natural aloe in the autoimmune and gastrointestinal areas of medicine. Additional researchers have now proven that these long-chain polysaccharides can indeed improve severe systems of intestinal disorders. Could the aloe plant have the medical properties to heal Crohn's disease?

The aloe plant formulation is exactly what cured my daughter of this monster disease. The specific treatment that we chose was AMP Floracel, a proven aloe formulation. AMP Floracel gave Kelly her life back. I am so positive that this product will also work for you that on behalf of all my readers suffering with Crohn's disease, I have talked to CCH Nutrition Corp to let them know you will be calling for the same AMP Floracel that cured my daughter Kelly. Below is the contact information for CCH Nutrition Corp:

CCH Nutrition Corp
1314 E Las Olas Blvd
Fort Lauderdale FL 33301
Phone: 866-775-3332
Web site: http://ampforacel.com

AMP FLORACEL—OUR MIRACLE CURE

AMP Floracel is an aloe plant formulation that is 100 percent all natural and non-toxic. It has no side effects and can be taken with any other prescription medication as well as natural supplements.

AMP Floracel works inside your digestive tract. It's like when you have a burn on your skin and you apply aloe to heal the burned area. The product works in the same way only in your digestive tract. It coats your intestines so that everything flows smoothly. This is where the healing process begins. It will distribute the nutrients throughout your body and help boost and restore your immune system.

AMP Floracel Properties:

- Is 100% non-toxic with no negative side effects.
- Is 100% natural and available in capsule form.
- May be used simultaneously with any medication.
- Normalizes an array of damaging processes in the digestive tract.
- Is not digested by the enzyme systems—it is taken up into the cell intact.
- Promotes proliferation of healthy flora in the digestive tract.
- Fuels all bodily systems through the promotion of proper digestion, absorption, and assimilation of foods and nutrients
- Is absorbed through special receptor sites which exist within the human digestive tract.
- Stops the bleeding, damage, and leakage of the intestine wall, thereby taking the stress off the immune system.
- Effectively balances and restores proper immune system function.
- Acts as a potent anti-inflammatory agent to reduce inflammation.

- Increases circulation throughout the body and aids in blood-sugar balancing.
- Promotes and accelerates the tissue healing process.
- Rebuilds the intestinal protective mucosa lining.
- Controls chronic yeast growth so that normal, healthy flora may thrive.
- Permeates every cell in the body.
- Has direct anti-bacterial, anti-viral, anti-fungal, anti-yeast, and anti-parasitic effects.
- Contributes greatly to prevention and healing of malignant cells.
- Is an extremely effective intracellular antioxidant and free-radical scavenger.
- Increases phagocytes dramatically to ingest foreign viral and bacterial agents.
- Eliminates mal-digestion and thus a host of pathological reactions.

Common knowledge among many researchers is that the body's natural mechanism against disease (the immune system) is highly dependent upon the absorption of nutrients to fuel its function. It is crucial to have the proper absorption of the essential nutrients. Without balanced nutrients, the immune system is unable to fight off potential disease or to effectively fight against existing conditions. In other words, the body's ability to fight off potential disease or to recover from disease without essential nutrients is, for the most part, impossible. Nutrients are a very important key to recovery, and the body must be capable of absorbing them. You can read more about AMP Floracel, including more testimonials like the ones on the back cover, an ABC News story, and actual doctors opinions, at ampfloracel.com

OTHER ALTERNATIVE TREATMENTS THAT I RESEARCHED AND DOCUMENTED:

PEPPERMINT OIL

Peppermint oil may relieve some common symptoms of irritable bowel syndrome. The oil travels to the small and large intestines where it relaxes intestinal muscles, thereby relieving symptoms. Peppermint oil should be taken in capsule or coated pills form to prevent it from being released directly in the stomach. It is important to know that in the stomach, peppermint oil can cause heartburn by relaxing the sphincter muscles that separate the stomach from the esophagus, allowing a reflux of acid from the stomach into the esophagus, which is why the capsules are coated to prevent them from melting in the stomach. You should not use peppermint oil in its pure form for this reason. You can purchase peppermint oil capsules at most health-food stores.

FISH OIL

Fish oil has an anti-inflammatory effect similar to corticosteroids and aspirin without the side effects and at very little cost in capsule form. The element in fish oil that cools down or neutralizes inflammatory, disease-producing prostaglandins and leukotrienes is called Omega-3 fatty acid. Studies have proven that fish oil supplements reduce inflammation in the colon by 60 percent. Examinations by sigmoidoscopy revealed less inflammation or damage to patients who use fish oil supplements as opposed to those who did not include fish oil in their diet. It has also been proven that some patients were able to cut their dosage of prednisone in half. Italian doctors have started using fish oil supplements to prolong remission in Crohn's patients. Fish is an exceedingly remarkable therapeutic and preventive food with enormous curing powers.

ST. JOHN'S WORT

St John's Wort eases anxiety by acting as a mild tranquilizer and antidepressant. It lowers levels of the brain chemical monoamine oxidase (MAO). The theory is that St John's Wort helps in reducing stress that may elevate the severity of intestinal diseases. Studies have shown adverse effects and drug interactions with St John's Wort. The most common adverse effects reported are dizziness, confusion, and tiredness. Drug interactions with St John's Wort have shown to decrease the concentration and effect of some prescription medications.

OLIVE OIL

Olive oil has been used for centuries as an all-purpose miracle remedy. The benefits of using olive oil for Crohn's patients are many; this simple oil has been proven to loosen the bowels, stimulate bile flow, soothe intestinal mucus membranes, and restore damaged tissue. The active ingredient oleic acid has been proven to block chemicals in the bowel that aggravate Crohn's inflammation, allowing the body to heal. Olive oil also contains a wide variety of valuable antioxidants believed to play a major role in the wide range of health benefits. Two to three tablespoons of olive oil per day are suggested to maximize these health benefits. Extra virgin olive oil contains the most potent, disease fighting chemicals. Olive oil therapy can be added to your current Crohn's medical treatment with confidence as there are no drug interactions or adverse reactions documented.

MAGNESIUM CITRATE

For extreme constipation, magnesium citrate works wonders. This little secret medication can be bought without a prescription from your local pharmacy or retail store. Magnesium citrate absorbs increased water into your intestines which causes peristalsis to occur. Peristalsis is a wavelike motion which moves fecal matter through your intestines. Since your intestines will be absorbing this excess water from your body it is very important to drink plenty of water after taking magnesium citrate to keep from becoming dehydrated.

WORMS

New studies and research are currently being done on the positive effects that worms have inside the bowel. The theory is that the worm eggs hatch inside the bowel, helping to restore mucus production and suppressing the body's immune response, which lessens inflammation. More research is needed, and if you are interested in worm therapy, it is advised that you discuss with your doctor your possibilities of being part of a clinical trial study.

CAT'S CLAW

Cat's claw is an herbal product that has anti-inflammatory properties and the ability to fight certain viruses. Studies have shown adverse effects and drug interactions. Drug interactions have shown to decrease the concentration and effect of some prescription medications.

FEEL GOOD TIP AND HELPFUL HINTS:

HEAT

Heating pads are a great source of relaxation for those aching muscles, but be cautious when sleeping with these as they can burn your skin. Purchase a heating pad with an automatic shut off if you intend to sleep with one. For daily heat, the 8-hour heating patches are great for lower back and lower stomach discomfort. At the end of a trying day, take time to treat yourself to a relaxing hot bath. A hot bath will ease some of those aches and pains associated with Crohn's disease.

Add a little Epsom salt to enhance your soak. However, go light on the Epsom salt as it is absorbed through the skin, and too much Epsom salt in your system may not be well tolerated and could lead to adverse effects such as dehydration.

BATHROOM TIPS

Crohn's suffers spend a lot of time in the Bathroom, so make it a room that is as bright and comfy as possible. Maybe a new coat of paint in a relaxing color is needed, or a new inspirational shower curtain. Hang motivating pictures or family photos on the walls and don't forget the cushion toilet seat. Get creative and make your bathroom a calming place to be.

The Caveman Position

As a Crohn's suffer you may have loose stool one day and hard painful stool the next day. For those hard stool days, the Caveman Position, as Kelly called it, may help. With your back straight raise your knees up as close to your chest as you can, flex and release your back muscles. Repeat the flexing of the back muscles as often as needed. This position seems to relieve some of the pressure and pain associated with hard stool movement and the flexing helps get the colon moving.

CONSTIPATION VS DIARRHEA

The Colon Wars: Constipation vs Diarrhea. This seems to be a daily occurrence when battling this monster disease. When feeling the pain and bloating of mild constipation, a pre-bottled, disposable sodium phosphate enema solution is available over the counter and may help. These single use bottles come pre-lubricated for a safe and relaxing insertion. When administrating the solution, lie on your left side, try to relax and administer slowly. If immediate relief is not needed than Metamucil has the same effects on the colon and comes in oral pill form. For mild to moderate diarrhea, over the counter anti-diarrhea medication can be taken.

MASSAGE

The only advantage to having Crohn's disease is the excuse to have regularly scheduled body and back massages. Ask your massage technician to concentrate on the lower back and left side of the back, which may help to keep the colon from becoming impacted. Relax and enjoy.

EARLY TO BED, EARLY TO RISE...

While your body sleeps it is healing itself, so don't feel guilty about turning in early. Make it a habit to wake up early enough to have time for your bathroom needs, eliminating the stress of feeling rushed.

CLOSING THOUGHT

I do know personally the effects that this monster disease has on a loved one, the long days of depression, pain and hopelessness that they endure. If you are caring for a loved one diagnosed with Crohn's disease, it is important to keep a positive attitude and never give up hope that together you will beat this disease. If you are suffering from Crohn's disease, don't let a bad day get you down. At the end of the day, go to bed with a positive look forward. "Tomorrow will be a better day." Say it out loud, over and over, until you believe it! A positive attitude and perseverance are your secret weapons in battling this monster. Your doctor may have suggested, as they did to Kelly, that the road ahead will be long and hopeless, but it is up to you to pave your road with fortitude, hope, and your dreams of a healthier tomorrow. I pray that you find the miracle cure that will rid your body of this monstrous disease.

SOURCES

About Crohn's Disease. (2009). Available at http://www. ccfa.org/info/about/crohns.

Crohn's disease. From Mayo Foundation for Medical Education and Research.(2010). Available at: http://www.mayoclinic.com/health/crohns-disease/ DS00104.

NIH Publication No. 06-3410. From National Digestive Diseases Information Clearinghouse. (2006). Available at: http://digestive.niddk.nih.gov/ddiseases/pubs/ crohns/1.NIH

Living with Crohn's Disease. (2009). Available at: http:// www.ccfa.org/frameviewer/?url=/media/pdf/ crohns2005.pdf.

Crohn's Disease and FoodResources for Living with Crohn's Disease. Visit and learn more now. www.CrohnsOnline. com/Diet

Wikipedia, www.Wikipedia.org

Miracle Food Cures from the Bible, 1999, Prentice Hall

Everhart, JE, ed. *The Burden of Digestive Disease in the United States.* Bethesda, MD: National Institute of Diabetes and Digestive and Kidney Diseases, US Dept. of Health and Human Services; 2008 NIH publication 09-6433

Mayo Clinic, "Crohn's Disease"

National Digestive Diseases Information Clearinghouse

1998-2011 Mayo Foundation for Medical Education and Research.

AMP Floracel : ampfloracel.com